THE LITTLE BOOK ABOUT

SEX

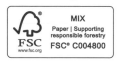

Published in 2023 by OH!
An Imprint of Welbeck Non-Fiction Limited,
part of Welbeck Publishing Group.
Offices in London – 20 Mortimer Street, London W1T 3JW
and Sydney – Level 17, 207 Kent St, Sydney NSW 2000 Australia
www.welbeckpublishing.com

Compilation text © Welbeck Non-Fiction Limited 2023
Design © Welbeck Non-Fiction Limited 2023

ISBN 978-1-80069-547-4

Written and compiled by: Malcolm Croft
Editorial: Victoria Denne
Project manager: Russell Porter
Design: Tony Seddon
Production: Jess Brisley

A CIP catalogue record for this book is available from the British Library

Printed in Dubai

10 9 8 7 6 5 4 3 2 1

THE LITTLE BOOK ABOUT

SEX

EVERYTHING
YOU EVER WANTED
TO GOOGLE
ABOUT SEX WITHOUT
HAVING TO
DELETE YOUR
BROWSING HISTORY

CONTENTS

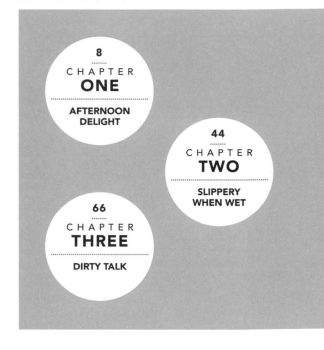

INTRODUCTION

Sex has been on the mind of every resident of Earth since the first penetrative copulation 385 million years ago, by fish nonetheless! With the appearance of our distant cousins, and originators of the first double entendre, *Homo erectus*, sex went from perfunctory procreation to an extremely fetishized sport for enjoyment. As the great Lily Tomlin said, "Man first walked upright simply to free his hands for masturbation."

However, it is only in the last century, if that, that humans have even begun to understand what sex is, let alone harness its beauty and power. Where it was once kept in a closet with the lights out, the mucky little secret everybody whispered about, now most parts of the world have run amok with it, turning its tricks on every part of the human anatomy. Indeed, when it comes to sex, every hole's a goal.

Welcome, then, to *The Little Book About Sex*, a journey into the delightful world of sex, relationships and everything bedroom related! This is everything you ever wanted to Google about the saucy subject without having to delete your browser history afterwards. From the awkward encounters that make you cringe to the hilarious mishaps that leave you in stitches, this book captures the hilarity that often accompanies the matters of the heart and the bedroom. With a blend of witty facts, hilarious quotes and what we like to call playful observations, this little book will have you giggling and nodding in recognition.

So, whether you're a love guru or a newbie to the dating scene, *The Little Book About Sex* is the perfect companion for both singles and couples alike. All you've got to do to enjoy the wild ride is turn over and try to enjoy yourself!

CHAPTER
ONE

AFTERNOON DELIGHT

Welcome to the pleasure dome, the breeding ground of carnal knowledge! There are so many nooks and crannies to poke our noses into that we should probably get on with it before we over-excite ourselves and fall asleep.

Who's up for a spot of afternoon delight?

> **"**
> Everything in the world
> is about sex, except sex.
> Sex is about power.
> **"**

Oscar Wilde

Cunnilingo No.1

Procasturbating – Masturbating to defeat boredom, or kill time.

Doppelbanger – Sex with someone that looks identical to you (but isn't actually related).

Shrimping – Orgasm-inducing toe suckage.

Mastuwaiting – A phrase that defines a porn video's buffering midway through masturbation.

Nooner – A sexual encounter just before lunchtime.

In France, the famous term for orgasm is *la petite mort*, or "the little death". The expression describes the post-orgasm euphoric sensation that feels like a brief loss of consciousness.

The French also say *voir les anges*, which translates to "seeing the angels", which is much more divine.

66

God gave men both a penis and a brain, but unfortunately not enough blood supply to run both at the same time.

99

Robin Williams

Love Language: French

While English distracted itself with puerile slang, the French kept sex sexy with incredibly elegant-sounding euphemisms.

Une partie de jambes en l'air
(Apart with your legs in the air)

Tailler une pipe
(Cut a blowjob)

Descendre à la cave
(Descend into a cave)
To perform oral sex on a woman

Avoir du monde au balcon
(To have lots of people on the balcony)
Big breasts

Tremper son biscuit
(To dip his cookie)
Promiscuous

Planter la tente
(To set up the tent)
To get an erection

Va te faire foutre
(Go make yourself ejaculate)
Fuck off

Voulez vous coucher avec moi?
(Do you want to sleep with me?)

Rub and Tug

History is stuffed with slang for masturbation. These are our favourites. Which one do you use?

MALE	FEMALE
Cuffing the Carrot	Buffin' the Muffin
Beating the Bishop	Flicking the Bean
Burping the Worm	Debugging the Hard Drive
Choking the Chicken	Poaching the Egg
Charming the Cobra	Double-Clicking the Mouse
Making the Bald Man Cry	Petting the Cat
Spanking the Monkey	Rubbin' the Nubbin
Pocket Hockey	Pinball
Jacking the Beanstalk	Manual Override
Playing the Skin Flute	Finger Painting
Shaking Hands With the Milkman	Primin' the Hymen
Polishing the Banister	Riding the Unicycle
Strangling the Swan	Ménage à Moi

According to a Healthline survey, women's ideal foreplay duration is 20 minutes. Men, on average, devote 5–10 minutes to foreplay.

For women, a desirable amount of intercourse would last between 7–13 minutes.

"
Sex without love is
as hollow and ridiculous
as love without sex.
"

Hunter S Thompson

8,000

The amount of nerve endings in a clitoris – twice as many as a penis. In fact, most of the nerve endings that contribute to the female orgasm are on the surface of the vulva and do not require penetration to be stimulated to orgasm.

In Japanese,
female masturbation is called
shiko shiko manzuri, or
"10,000 rubs".

Its male counterpart, *senzuri*,
means "A thousand rubs".

Penis

Derived from the Latin word
for tail, *pēnis*, which emerged
from the Greek translation of
phallus, meaning "to swell" –
a tail that swells.

Wanking Around the World

Aftrekken – Tear It Off – Dutch

Zsebhoki – Pocket Hockey – Hungarian

Runka – To Wobble – Swedish

Ditalino – Small Thimble (Fingering) – Italian

Echando Paja – Throwing Hay – Venezuelan

Litbol Et Ha Vafle – To Soak the Waffle – Hebrew

Jalarla – To Pull It – Spanish

Nappe Laksen – Tugging the Salmon – Swedish

Cinco Contra Um – Five Against One – Portuguese

Bić Niemca – To Punch a German – Polish

Stiskanje Guje – To Squeeze the Viper – Croatian

Descabelar O Palhaço – To Tousle the Clown – Brazilian Portuguese

Lysogo V Kulake Gonyat – To Pet One's Monkey – Russia

Foreplaylist: Classic Pop

"Sexual Healing" – Marvin Gaye

"I Want a Little Sugar In My Bowl" – Nina Simone

"Wicked Game" – Chris Isaak

"Sexy M.F." – Prince

"I'm Gonna Love You Just a Little More Babe" – Barry White

"The Sweetest Taboo" – Sade

"Lady Marmalade" – Labelle

"Love to Love You Baby" – Donna Summer

"I Just Wanna Make Love to You" – Etta James

"Je t'Aime...Moi Non Plus" – Serge Gainsbourg

"Feel Like Makin' Love" – Roberta Flack

The first dictionary for sex was Copland's *Hye Waye*, published circa 1535. The trendy word of the day to mean sexual intercourse back then was *dock*, a penis was an *instrument* and an erection was a *stand*.

Callet, *drab* and *dell* all meant whore, of which there were a lot back then.

Fifty Shades of Grey by E. L. James is the world's No.1 bestselling erotic fiction book series, sometimes referred to as "cliterature". The series has now sold over 150 million copies worldwide. UK sex toy retailer Lovehoney saw a 68 per cent rise in profits following the first book's publication!

In a recent study by Durex,

67 per cent

of women claim they've faked
an orgasm more than once.

61 per cent do so in order for
the sex to finish faster.

11 per cent

The percentage of men
aged 16–74 in the UK that
have paid for sex on at least
one occasion – roughy
2.3 million individuals.

35,000

Cuban dictator Fidel Castro takes the worldwide top-spot, it is believed, for the most shag-happy man. For more than four decades, Castro reportedly had sex with two women a day – one for lunch and one for dinner.

1922

The first ever erotic kiss between two lesbian women in a Hollywood film was in Cecil B. DeMille's 1922 motion picture, *Manslaughter*.

44 per cent

The percentage of men, on average, who have exaggerated their number of sexual partners.

28 per cent

The percentage of
Americans who believe
sex before marriage is
morally unacceptable.

The Great British public
have the most sexual partners
compared to its European
cousins, averaging seven
lifetime sexual partners.

The European average is 6.2.

Louisiana is the U.S. state that loves sex the most, based on sexual partner data.

The Pelican State averaged 15.7 partners – six times more sexual partners than the residents of Utah, America's least sexual place with an average of 2.6.

91 per cent

The percentage of men who prefer a woman to initiate foreplay.

7.5

From a recent Durex study, the figure both sexes agreed, on average, was the ideal number of sexual partners in a lifetime.

According to the BBC, 385 million years ago, fish known as *Microbrachius dicki* (seriously) were the first-known creature to reproduce by sex, not spawning. This primitive, 8cm-long bony fish lived in lakes, predominately in what is now Scotland.

"They couldn't have done it in a 'missionary position'," said Professor Long, their discoverer. "The very first act of copulation was done sideways, square-dance style."

Hotline Bling

A millennial's term for a booty call (not to be confused with a butt dial).

The phrase became popular after the chart-topping 2015 song, "Hotline Bling" by U.S. rapper, Drake.

"

We are all born sexual creatures, thank God, but it's a pity so many people despise and crush this natural gift.

"

Marilyn Monroe

In a 2017 study by the Kinsey Institute, it was revealed that lesbians orgasm 86 per cent of the time during sex, compared to 65 per cent for straight women.

The same report concluded that straight men orgasmed 95 per cent of the time.

1 in 5

The number of lesbian women,
according to a recent survey
by AutoStraddle, who orgasm
multiple times during sex.

The verb *fuck* was first recorded in 1508 in William Dunbar's poem "In Secreit Place this Hyndir Nycht". Contrary to popular legend, "fuck" does not originate from the acronym F.U.C.K. (Fornication Under Command of the King), rather from the Germanic word *fricken*, to hit.

Lesbian Sex Positions to Write Home About

According to *Cosmopolitan*, the ten best lesbian sex positions for "truly mind-blowing orgasms" are below. Off you go! (You'll have to Google them for instructions.)

1. The Slider

2. The Made to Order

3. The Bumper Cars

4. The Daily Grind

5. The Double Trouble

6. The Laconic Lounger

7. The All-Hands Meeting

8. The Rocket

9. The Kinky Jockey

10. Defying Gravity

October 21, 1992

The day the world's biggest star published her infamous *Sex* book – stufffed with 128 pages of erotica, nudity and semi-sexually explicit images and fantasies written by Madonna. In today's world it would be considered tame but back then it was the height of scandal.

CHAPTER
TWO

SLIPPERY WHEN WET

Sex is often best enjoyed with a companion. So, take our hand, and let's dip our digits in and out of arousal's bliss-filled abyss with more sextistics, quotes and throbbing facts than a dominatrix can shake her leather whip at. Don't forget to sign your consent waiver, things are about to get wet 'n' wild...

69

This naughty numerical slang is French, of course. It had to be. It dates back to the French Revolution. It was first used in a 1790 publication, *The Whore's Catechisms*, written by revolutionary figure Théroigne de Méricour, who described a *soixante-neuf*, or

69, as the ideal post-cursor to fine wine and a dining, two other things the French famously taught the world.

The sexual position was described in the *Kama Sutra* as the Congress of a Crow. It slipped its way into English a century later, circa the 1880s.

138

The world record for female orgasms in one hour.*

*16 is the world record for male orgasms in one hour. Unbeatable, right?

In 1966, as part of a
scientific experiment, a
woman enjoyed a

45-second orgasm

that involved 25 individual
contractions, officially the
longest orgasm ever recorded
in one sitting.

13.5 inches (34 cm)

The largest officially recorded human penis, when fully erect, belongs to New Yorker Jonah Falcon. Flaccid, this member dangles at 9.5 inches (24 cm).

919

The number of sex partners American adult film actress Lisa Sparxxx had in a 12-hour period in 2004, a world record, as part of an EroticCon stunt.

Each man was permitted 45 seconds.

Refractory Period

The period of time between male orgasms before they will be able to feel sexually aroused again.*

*Teenage males have a refractory period of about 15 minutes. Men in their seventies can take 20 hours. The average for all men is half an hour.

Cocktail: Sex on the Beach

The world's sexiest cocktail.

Ingredients

50 ml vodka

25 ml peach schnapps

2 oranges, juiced + 2 slices to garnish

50 ml cranberry Juice

Glacé cherries, to garnish (optional)

Ice

Do It Right

Lube up two tall glasses with a dunk of two large ice cubes. Then pour the vodka, peach schnapps and fruit juices into a large jug. Stir until mixed. Pour equally into the two glasses and stir seductively to mix. Pop a cherry and orange slice on top for half-time refreshment.

The very first (non-pornographic) sex scene on the silver screen cinema was in the 1933 erotic drama *Ekstase* by Czech director Gustav Machatý.

It was the first film to feature an actor, 18-year-old Hedy Lamarr, perform an orgasm onscreen. Lamarr would soon become an icon of Hollywood's golden age.

"

Oooh, Oh, Ooh, Ooh, Oh
God, Ooh, Oh God, Oh, Oh,
Oh, Oh God, Oh Yeah Right
There, Oh, Oh, Oh, Oh, Oh
God, Oh, Yes! Yes! Yes! Yes!
Yes! Yes! Ah, Ah, Oh Yes! Yes!
Yes! Oh, Yes! Yes! Yes! Yes! Yes!
Yes! Oh, Oh, Oh, Oh God, Oh.

"

Meg Ryan's infamous big-screen orgasm
in 1989's *When Harry Met Sally*. The diner scene
climaxes with the famous line of a nearby customer:
"I'll have what she's having."

Grape
Maraschino cherries
Tomato
Strawberry
Cough syrup
Pasta
Jelly
Chilli
Milk
Sparkling water
Honey

In order of consumption, in the infamous erotic film
9½ Weeks (1988), the food in the legendary sex scene,
featuring Mickey Rourke and Kim Basinger. Serving
suggestions were not given.

66

For women, the best
aphrodisiacs are words.
The G-spot is in the ears.
He who looks for it below
there is wasting his time.

99

Isabel Allende

In a 2022 survey conducted by Lloyds Pharmacy, the top 20 most-used euphemisms in the regions of the UK:

East	**Pussy**
East Midlands	**Foo Foo**
London	**Vajayjay**
North East	**Foof**
North West	**Fanny**
Northern Ireland	**Nunny**
Scotland	**Private Parts**
South East	**Minge**
South West	**Noo Noo**
Wales	**Lady Bits**
West Midlands	**Down There**
Yorkshire and the Humber	**Vag**

45 per cent

The number of males in the UK who think they have a small penis.

**2.8 to 3.9 inches
(7 to 10 centimetres)**
Average length of a flaccid
penis in the UK.

**4.7 to 6.3 inches
(12 to 16 centimetres)**
Average length of an erect
penis in the UK.

Vagina

Derived from the Latin for "sheath", a long, tight-fitting case for the blade of a sword.

Clitoris

Derived from the Late Greek word *kleitoris*, to mean both "little hill" and "to rub".

The clitoris is so much more than a pea-sized nub to rub, however. Like icebergs, 90 per cent of a clitoris' majesty lies beneath the surface.

Hysteria

Hysteria is literally translated from the Greek term for "suffering in the uterus" – *hysterika*. In the sexually repressed Victorian Age (1820–1914), it was believed a quarter of women suffered from medical symptoms of "hysteria", including sexual desire and excessive vaginal wetness.

It wasn't until 1952 that "hysteria" as a medical diagnosis was abandoned following the obvious realization that female arousal and sexual pleasure were normal and healthy.

66

Nymphomaniac: a woman as obsessed with sex as an average man.

99

Mignon McLaughlin

66

A man can sleep around, no questions asked, but if a woman makes nineteen or twenty mistakes she's a tramp.

99

Joan Rivers

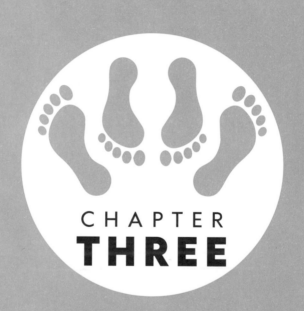

CHAPTER
THREE

DIRTY TALK

Now that we've scratched the surface
of sex, it's time to dive down deeper into its
darkest dwellings.

From masturbation to BDSM, and everything
in-between (which is a lot), there's no sex
too taboo for this tiny tome of trivia. Let's talk
about sex, baby...

It was U.S. scientist Alfred Kinsey, and founder of the Kinsey Institute in 1947, who carried out huge sexual surveys in the 1940s that first scientifically demystified the sexual behaviour of males and females, the female orgasm, and masturbation. He is renowned as the "father of the sexual revolution".

Today, the Kinsey Institute is the trusted source for critical issues in sexuality, gender and reproduction.

Orgasm

Derived from the Greek
orgasmos, to mean
"excitement" and "swelling".

A man will typically spend 20 seconds a week, 12 minutes a year, and 10 hours in a typical lifetime in the throes of orgasm.

One of the first invented vibrators was released in 1891. It was called the "Manipulator" and was powered by steam.

It was so loud to operate that not even your lover could hear you scream.

Regardless, it was a big hit.

In the early 1880s, British doctor Joseph Mortimer Granville invented the first electromechanical vibrator by mistake.

It was originally invented to relieve aching back muscles. It would become the fifth home appliance to benefit from electricity, after the toaster, fan, kettle and sewing machine.

"

Graze on my lips; and if those hills be dry, stray lower, where the pleasant fountains lie.

"

William Shakespeare

0.1 mm

The diameter of an ovum.
This is 30 times larger than
the length of a sperm, which
measures $\frac{1}{500}$ of an inch.

100 million

The average number of sperm in an ejaculation. In their testes, men produce 1,500 sperm per second. Only three per cent of semen contains sperm cells and only a few hundred actually reach the ovum.

10 Steps to Better Sex

(according to *The Guardian*, so this could all be wrong. Anyway...)

1. Create a safe and comfortable environment.

2. Turn off your phone.

3. Be curious and playful with your touch.

4. Vary movements in classic sex positions; don't try anything too acrobatic for the sake of it.

5. Don't wait until the end of the day. Afternoon sex is the best.

6. Don't chase a female orgasm. And penis ejaculation doesn't have to be the end.

7. Lube up to heighten the sensations.

8. Masturbation in a relationship is healthy and should be encouraged, even shared.

9. It's OK to admit that sex can be a chore. Remember, sexual desire ebbs and flows.

10. Focus on what you both want out of sex, not what should happen.

66

My wife is a sex
object – every time I ask
for sex, she objects.

99

Les Dawson

10 Things to Think of to Slow Down Ejaculation

1. The plot of *Inception*.

2. Your partner's grandmother in her underwear (particularly if she's dead).

3. An unfinished and overdue work project.

4. That time you broke your leg.

5. Your favourite track from your favourite album and why.

6. How to cook the perfect steak.

7. The concept of time and the infinite void of the universe.

8. All the ways in which you're turning into your dad.

9. The player line-ups of two teams in any sporting event.

10. Your mother's face in orgasm mode.

The world is having less sex.

The British National Surveys of Sexual Attitudes has concluded that the average number of occasions of sex per week has decreased with each decade and is an international trend. In 1991, the average was five times a month. In 2021, the average was two times a month.

75 per cent of modern couples cite work schedules and hectic social lives as the primary reason for a decreased interest in sex.

In the Victorian Era,
the Greek word "orgasm"
was considered too lewd for a
repressed society.

Paroxysms, a word to mean a
"sudden outburst of emotion",
was deemed more appropriate.

The Greek god of marriage, and son of Apollo, was Hymen. He died on his wedding night and by doing so lent his name to the thin membrane that covers the vaginal opening, which supposedly was to be broken during sexual intercourse on the first night of a virgin woman's marriage.

Why Don't We Do It In the Road?

The ten riskiest places Americans admitted they've had sex, according to a survey by EdenFantasys.com. It's your job to put them in order of risk...

1. Fast-Food Drive-Thru

2. Boss's Desk

3. Dentist's Chair

4. While Driving 70 mph Down a Highway

5. Top of the Empire State Building

6. On a Train Track

7. Courthouse Bathroom

8. Inside a Haunted House Attraction

9. New York City Subway

10. Dean's Office at University

Top Ten Things Most Said in Bed

"God." / "Jesus."

"Fuck." / "Yes." / "Baby."

"Harder." / "Deeper."

"Just like that."

"That feels so good."

"I'm so hard for you right now."

"I'm gonna cum."

"Is it OK?"

"I want you inside me."

"I've thought about this all day."

According to Durex's Global Sexual Well-Being Survey, the top 10 nations who have the most sex are as follows. Percentages indicate the number of adults who have sex at least once a week.

1. Greece: *87 per cent**

2. Brazil: *82 per cent*

3. Russia: *80 per cent*

4. China: *78 per cent*

5. Italy: *76 per cent*

6. Poland: *76 per cent*

7. Malaysia: *74 per cent*

8. Switzerland: *72 per cent*

9. Spain: *72 per cent*

10. Mexico: *71 per cent*

*Hardly a surprise. It was the Greeks who gave the world aphrodisiacs, eroticism, narcissism and nymphomania.

According to Durex's Global Well-Being Survey, the top 10 most sexually satisfied countries are as follows.

1. Nigeria: *67 per cent*
2. Mexico: *63 per cent*
3. India: *61 per cent*
4. Poland : *54 per cent*
5. Greece: *51 per cent*
6. Holland: *50 per cent*
7. South Africa: *50 per cent*
8. Spain: *49 per cent*
9. Canada : *48 per cent*
10. USA: *48 per cent*

Sexual satisfaction is defined as free from stress, ability to orgasm, free from sexual dysfunction and frequency of sex and foreplay. Percentages indicate the number of adults who have sex at least once a week.

According to Durex's Global Well-Being Survey, the top 10 countries that have the least amount of sex in a year on average are as follows:

1. Japan: *45* times per year
2. Singapore: *73* times per year
3. India: *75* times per year
4. Indonesia: *77* times per year
5. Hong Kong: *78* times per year
6. Malaysia: *83* times per year
7. Vietnam: *87* times per year
8. Taiwan: *88* times per year
9. Sweden: *92* times per year
10. China: *96* times per year

> **"**
> Life is like sex.
> It's not always good, but
> it's always worth trying.
> **"**

Pamela Anderson

The *Kama Sutra*, an ancient Indian text written in Sanskrit between 400 BCE and 300 CE, is much more than the original manual on sex positions. The text celebrates the art and nature of love and living well, finding a partner and maintaining a healthy pleasurable sex life.

Well worth a read. Five stars.

66

Take me to bed or lose me forever.

99

Carole (Meg Ryan), *Top Gun* (1986)

66
I did not have sexual relations with that woman, Ms Lewinsky.
99
(Lie)

In 1988, President Bill Clinton and intern Monica Lewinsky had an affair inside the White House. It was the biggest sex scandal of the century. Famously, Lewinsky gave Clinton a blowjob in the Oval Office, which helped to "manage his anxieties", but also redefined the question: What is sex?

(Sex is defined as physical activity between two people in which they touch each other's sexual organs, and which may include sexual intercourse.)

50 per cent

The percentage of the U.S. population that has tried some form of BDSM – Bondage and Discipline, Dominance and Submission, Sadism and Masochism.

76 per cent

The percentage of men who get turned on by verbal reassurance that they're doing a good job in bed.

In 2014, the phrase "Netflix and Chill" was taken hostage by Gen Z to now mean "inviting a friend over for casual sex".

For married couples with children, "Netflix and Chill" is a new type of sex, not a euphemism.

74 per cent

The percentage of people whose favourite post-sex activity is a good old-fashioned cuddle.

According to the Royal Society Open Science, it takes men

5.4 minutes

to orgasm. This is the result of roughly 250 thrusts, or 50 pumps per minute.

62 per cent

The number of millennials who send sexts at least once a month. 48 per cent do it at least once a week.

Top Six Sex Fantasies in the U.S.

Having a threesome – 89 per cent of men want one.

BDSM – 93 per cent of women want to be sexually dominated.

Public locations – 84 per cent of women had a public sex fantasy.

Voyeurism – 54 per cent of men want to be watched.

Partner sharing – 64 per cent of men.

Same-sex fantasies – 59 per cent of straight women fantasised about sex with other women.

25 per cent

The percentage of men
who have claimed to have
faked an orgasm.

14 minutes

The time it takes, on average, for a woman to reach orgasm during sex with her partner.

(It's four minutes with masturbation.)

Women's orgasms last from

20–40 seconds

on average.

Men's orgasms last on average
five seconds.

Both are as strong as the other.

76 per cent

of Americans have had sex
in the great outdoors.

£340,000 a year

The cost to the NHS of surgically removing objects that have gotten stuck up bottoms. The average "anal extraction" costs almost £850 per object.

CHAPTER
FOUR

STICKY
FINGERS

As you'll soon discover, sex has many
pseudonyms, each as ridiculous as the last.
Sex, too, comes in all shapes and sizes, speeds
and sounds, from blink-and-you-miss-it
foreplay to hurry-up-and-finish sore lay, earth-
shattering screams to awkward silences.

Like a snowflake, sex is never the same twice,
a unique moment never to be repeated. Let's
savour the flavour with a few saucy sips of
wicked wit and wisdom...

In 2022, the global sex-toy market was valued at $32.7 billion and is expected to increase to $52 billion a year by 2030. More than 60 million sex toys are sold every year.

Ejaculatory Reflex

An automatic body response a man can't control. Try taking a large, deep breath as you feel the urge to ejaculate and it should calm the moment, albeit momentarily.

66

The best sex education
for kids is when Daddy
pats Mommy on the
fanny when he comes
home from work.

99

William H. Masters

66

The only unnatural sex act is that which you cannot perform.

99

Alfred Kinsey

21

The number of calories* burned typically from sexual intercourse. We burn on average three to four calories per minute during sex.

*If you've worked up a hunger, a teaspoon of semen contains approx. five calories, FYI.

The Benefits of a Healthy Sex Life

Lower blood pressure

Better immune system

Better heart health, lower risk for heart disease

Improved self-esteem

Decreased depression and anxiety

Increased libido

Immediate, natural pain relief

Better sleep

In 2021, a Harvard University study encouraged men to ejaculate more than 21 times a month in order to reduce their prostate cancer risk by one-third.

In 2022,
163 million

Americans over 18 had purchased a sex toy.

(There are only 108 million females in this age range.)

46.3 per cent*

The percentage of women
in the U.S. who use vibrators
while masturbating.

*The number of U.S. men who claim they aren't
threatened by vibrators is 70 per cent.

According to historical legend, Egyptian ruler Cleopatra was one of the first owners of a vibrator. By vibrator, we mean, of course, a gourd filled with scores of pissed-off bees. Cleopatra, we assume, would place the buzzing gourd close to her genitals to aid stimulation.

19

According to Ohio University, the number of times young men, on average, think about sex per day. Young women reportedly averaged ten thoughts about sex per day.

Persistent Genital Arousal Disorder (PGAD) is a rare, but real, and unfortunate, condition. It can cause sufferers to endure hundreds of orgasms every day without any stimulation or desire.

Four hours

Consult your doctor if a natural erection lasts longer. Something's up.

Top 11 Most Promiscuous Nations, 2023

1. Finland
2. New Zealand
3. Slovenia
4. Lithuania
5. Austria
6. Latvia
7. Croatia
8. Israel
9. Bolivia
10. Argentina
11. United Kingdom

In 1996, two years before Viagra hit the market, Charles Lennon received a penile implant. It gave him the superpower to raise and lower his penis on command.

Unfortunately, the implant stopped working and his penis was stuck in erect mode for 10 years.

Lennon sued the company responsible in 2004 and was awarded $400,000 in compensation.

66

Sex is emotion in motion.

99

Mae West

G-Spot

Its existence, or lack thereof, is a source of controversy. What we do know is that it could have been called Whipple Tickle after Dr Beverley Whipple (who coined "G-Spot") if we'd all had a bit more of a sense of humour about sex.

1 in 200

The number of all sudden
deaths that sexual intercourse
is responsible for.

28 miles per hour

The average speed of semen when ejaculated from a penis, according to the Kinsey Institute.

Gymnophoria

The eerie sense that another person is mentally undressing you.

66

The difference between sex and love is I've never cum from love.

99

Amy Schumer

18.4 per cent

The percentage of women who can orgasm without direct clitoral stimulation.

13 Sex Positions to Google (and Oogle)

The Chairman	Golden Arch
Scoop Me Up	Valedictorian
The Spork	Stand and Deliver
Snow Angel	Upstanding Citizen
Standing Wheelbarrow	Butter Churner
The Good Ex	The Pretzel Dip
Cross Booty	

1/400

The number of men flexible enough to give themselves a blowjob. It's estimated, however, that all 400 have given it a try at some point.

66

Teeth placement and jaw stress and suction and gag reflex. And all the while bobbing up and down, moaning and trying to breathe through our noses. Easy? Honey, they don't call it a job for nothing.

99

Samantha Jones (Kim Cattrall), *Sex and the City*

Next time you see
a man in the pits of
toxic masculinity, just
remember his penis
started life as a clitoris.

The world's most popular sex positions, in order of preference (on average)

1. Doggy-style

2. Missionary

3. Cowgirl

4. Holding Legs Up

5. 69

6. Spooning

7. Reverse Cowgirl

66

Nose, vagina, butthole.
If God didn't want us to put
our fingers in there, why did
she make them perfectly
finger-sized?

99

Ilana Wexler (Ilana Glazer), *Broad City*

CHAPTER
FIVE

FUNNY BUSINESS

Sex is a funny old business, isn't it?

From the faces (and back muscles) we pull
to the noises we make and the liquids we lose,
there's nothing more hilarious than making
the beast with two backs.

If sex is God's way of playing a joke on
humans, it's a doozy, as these tasty tit-bits
of trivia attest...

10 Greatest Songs About Sex

Most songs are about sex, but these ones are the least subtle...

"Fuck the Pain Away" – Peaches
"Rocket" – Beyoncé
"Milkshake" – Kelis
"Touch of My Hand" – Britney Spears
"Dirrty" – Christina Aguilera ft. Redman
"Sex With Me" – Rihanna
"I Touch Myself" – The Divinyls
"Relax" – Frankie Goes To Hollywood
"2 Become 1" – Spice Girls
"Sexual Eruption" – Snoop Dogg

66

God created sex.
Priests created marriage.

99

Voltaire

66

May your penis hurt when you make love.

99

This was the curse found inscribed on a seventh-century lead tablet discovered by archaeologists in Cyprus, 2008. Nobody knows who wrote the curse, or why.

Cocktails: Blowjob

Ingredients

½ ounce amaretto liqueur

⅕ ounce Irish cream liqueur

Whipped cream, to top

Do It Right

Squirt the amaretto into the shot glass.
Dollop the Irish cream on top, pouring
it slowly over the back of a spoon.
Ejaculate the whipped cream on top;
don't mix. Neck it, then let your neck
feel caressed by its kiss.

37.5

The number of megabytes of DNA a single sperm delivers as its payload. A single ejaculation represents a data transfer of 15,875 gigabytes — the equivalent of a single man's pornography hard drive.

66

Love is a matter of
chemistry,
but sex is a matter
of physics.

99

Alexandre Dumas

Love Gods

Aphrodite – Greek goddess of sexual intercourse

Venus – Roman goddess of sexual intercourse

Kamadeva – Hindu god of human desire

Oshun – Yoruban goddess of pleasure, sexuality and fertility

Min – Egyptian god of reproduction, love, and sexual pleasure

Freyja – Norse goddess of love and sex

Tlazolteotl – Aztec goddess of lust, carnality and sexual misdeeds

Sex

Derived from the Latin *sexus* and French *sexe* and simply referred to genitals.

Origin: circa 1200.

It was not until the 19th century that sex was used to mean intercourse.

66

When it comes to sex,
the most important
six inches are the ones
between the ears.

Dr Ruth Westheimer

7 out of 10

The number of Americans, according to a 2021 study conducted by sex toy store EdenFantasys, who have had sex in a car.*

*The report didn't say whose car it was.

> **66**
>
> I swear to you
> I won't stop until
> your legs are shaking
> and the neighbours
> know my name.
>
> **99**

Horace Cope

Popular Sex Euphemisms Through the Centuries

Shaking of the Sheets – 1200s
Give a Girl a Green Gown – 1300s
Do the Deed of Darkness – 1500s
Make the Beast with Two Backs – 1500s
Amorous Congress – 1700s
Shoot Twixt Wind and Water – 1600s
Give One's Arse a Salad – 1600s
Grope for Trout in a Peculiar River – 1600s
Riding St George – 1800s
Have Your Corn Ground – 1800s
Horizontal Refreshment – 1800's
Make Whoopee – 1920s
A Roll in the Hay – 1940s

Orgasmo!

Worldwide ways to have an orgasm:

Gao Chao – "High Tide!" – Mandarin Chinese

Pracanda Uttējanā – "Drastic Excitement!" – Bengali

Nyt Mä Tulen – "I Am Fire!" – Finland

Ezra Shodan – "Satisfaction Is Happening!" – Persian

Cực Khoái – "Extreme Pleasure!" – Vietnam

Iku – "I'm Going!" – Japan

Konchayu – "I'm Ending!" – Russia

Už Budu – "I Will Be!" – Czech

66

The function of muscle is
to pull and not to push,
except in the case of the
genitals and the tongue.

99

Leonardo da Vinci

Acording to several "sexperts", the best time to have sex is 7:30 a.m., or roughly 45 minutes after waking up.

Morning sex, when our energy is at its highest, floods the body with endorphins that lowers blood pressure, reduces stress and puts us in the best mood possible to enjoy the day.

Pillow Talk

During orgasm, the region of your brain called the hypothalamus floods your body with the chemical oxytocin, the body's "love hormone", when sensory nerves in the skin and genitals are activated.

Unlike other hormones, oxytocin stimulates its own production. If the body is stressed, the release of oxytocin is blocked.

66

You think homosexuality is disgusting? Then, it follows as the night the day, that you find sex disgusting, for there is nothing done between two men or two women that is, by any objective standard, different from that which is done between a man and a woman.

99

Stephen Fry

66

Women who love women
are lesbians. Men,
because they can only
think of women in sexual
terms, define lesbian as
sex between women.

99

Rita Mae Brown

10 per cent

According to the National Institutes of Health, the number of heterosexual couples who regularly partake in a little anal sex.

66

There is nothing wrong
with going to bed with
someone of your own
sex. People should be very
free with sex, they should
draw the line at goats.

99

Elton John

Two million

The number of egg follicles a female is born with.

Only 450 will be released as eggs, following puberty.

Like sex itself, conception is not about who comes first; it's about the quality in general.

The biggest misconception is the fact that the fastest sperm to reach the egg is *not* the first the egg permits to enter. Using a system of biological mechanisms, the egg actively *chooses* the sperm it wants to be fertilized by. It lets only the right one in.

66

Sex is much better
with a woman,
but then one can't
live with a woman.

99

Marlene Dietrich

Diletto

The origin of the word "Dildo", from the Italian to mean "a woman's delight". Remember that the next time you call your husband a dildo.

200 per cent

The number by which the vaginal canal can expand from its normal size (three inches) during sexual arousal.

Globally, only three per cent of men have a penis longer than eight inches. The worldwide average length is 5.3 inches (13.58 cm).

One in ten dreams
is a sex dream.

33.44 million

The number of condoms
Americans bought in 2020,
during lockdown. You know,
the year when everyone
"worked" from home.*

*9.4 million of these were for Trojan Magnum condoms.

10 per cent

The percentage that the penis and vagina account as part of the body's erogenous zones.

The least touched zones of arousal on the body are: scalp, ears, naval, sacrum, armpits, wrists, fingertips and behind the knee.

A single ejaculation contains about five millimeters of sperm, or one tablespoon.*

*The required amount of blood to make a penis hard is two tablespoons.

In a study published in the *Archives of Sexual Behavior*, it was revealed that one of the main reasons humans have sex is not to make others feel good, but to boost their own self-esteem.

Sex gives us the confidence to feel powerful and more attractive.

8.38 billion

The size of the global condom market, in U.S. dollars, in 2022. It is projected to increase to 13 billion U.S. dollars by 2030. More than five billion condoms are sold every year worldwide.

"

Sex is a part of nature. I go along with nature.

"

Marilyn Monroe

Five years

How much younger you'll look when you have sex at least three times a week.

30 minutes

The average time it takes the fastest-swimming sperm to reach the ovum. The rest could take up to two days.

17

The age at which a man hits his
sexual peak.

35

The age at which a woman hits
her sexual peak.*

*God's playing a joke on us, isn't he?

Love Language: German

When it comes to whispering sweet nothings, the Germans could go on for days.

Die Möhre Schrubben – To Scrub One's Carrot

Bettgeflüster – Pillow Talk

Geschlechtsverkehr – Sexual Intercourse

Fleischpeitsche – Penis

Lustperle – Vagina

Morgenlatte – Morning Erection

Samenstau – Blue Balls

Schäferstündchen –
One-Night Stand

Fickstück – Fuckpiece

Deckhengst – Stud

Zweilochstute – Butt and Vagina Girl

Schwangerschaftsverhütungsmittel
– Contraception

Apart from sneezes, orgasms are the only other physiological response a human cannot voluntarily stop once it has started.

The most dangerous sex position is the Reverse Cowgirl. 50 per cent of hospital admissions for penile fractures occur in this position.

CHAPTER
SIX

ORGASMO!

We've climaxed together. Phew! Wasn't that fun? Short but sweet, but that's the way we like to do it.

At this post-orgasmic plateau, we bathe momentarily in the wet spot of happiness for a few more whispered sweet nothings before preparing ourselves for a few hours of cuddling... oh no, too late, we've fallen asleep.

You'll have to menage a moi this final chapter solo, but poke us if you need finishing off...

89 per cent

The percentage of couples that have come together at the same time during the course of their relationship.

However, on average, only 50 per cent of the times they have sex do they orgasm at the same time.

Cunnilingo No.2

Hotwifing – When partners offer up their significant other to outside partners as a matter of pride.

Wanxiety – The fear of thinking someone can see you masturbate.

Chore-play – House chores completed by partners that turn on their lover to the point of arousal.

Bonestorming – Having sex to clear your mind. (Like brainstorming, but using your genitals.)

Sexophobia

Genophobia – fear of sex

Rectophobia – fear of the rectum

Ithyphallophobia – fear of erections

Thelephobia – fear of nipples

Phallophobia – fear of male genitals

Spermatophobia – fear of sperm

Haphephobia – fear of human touch

Trypophobia – fear of holes

Coitophobia – fear of intercourse

Heterophobia – fear of the opposite sex

Nosophobia – fear of getting a disease or virus

Gymnophobia – fear of nudity

Like snowflakes and fingerprints, every woman's vagina is special. This is due to nerve endings being distributed in her genitalia uniquely to others. That means every woman needs to employ slightly different methods to achieve orgasm.

The pulsations a woman feels during orgasm are actually her uterus rocking back and forth trying to scoop up sperm that may have pooled at the back of the vagina to enhance fertility.

Lordosis Behaviour

Borrowed from the Greek word to mean "bent backward", *Lordosis*, in nature, is the act of a female creature presenting its genitals when it is receptive to sex.

Most mammals, including rodents, elephants and cats, display this behaviour. Worth a go!

Generation Sex

According to YouGov data:

Baby Boomers
Average of 10.7 sexual partners in their lifetime. Women 7.4 partners, Men 12.9.

Generation X
Average of 13.1 sexual partners in their lifetime. Women 10.1, Men 16.1.

Millennials
Average of 11.6 sexual partners in their lifetime. Women 10.8, Men 13.4.

Generation Z
An average of 5.6 sexual partners so far. Women 2.6, Men 7.6.

Safe Words

According to a 2020 survey conducted by the UK
sex toy brand Lovehoney, these are the most popular
safe words used during rough or experimental sex.

1. Red	**6.** Apple
2. Pineapple	**7.** Vanilla
3. Banana	**8.** Yellow
4. Orange	**9.** Blue
5. Peach	**10.** Unicorn

Which one do you use?

14 per cent

The percentage of people who
have had sex with one person
over the course of their life.

4 per cent

The percentage of people who don't know (or who have lost count) of their number of sexual partners.

Tribbing

The lesbian sex act of rubbing genitals together, akin to scissoring. The word originates from "tribadism", derived from the Greek *tribo*, meaning "to rub".

According to Columbia University, these are the defined bases for sex that have nothing to do with baseball. It's important to be clear on this:

First Base – kissing and French kissing

Second Base – breast and nipple play and petting above the waist

Third Base – stroking and oral stimulation of genitals

Home Run – sexual intercourse

Three Strikes – you're out!

Cataglottism

Also known as a French Kiss; a kiss with the tongues.*

*It's called a French Kiss, allegedly, because French women use more tongue when kissing, according to American WWII soldiers.

Sex drives reside in two areas of the brain: the cerebral cortex and the limbic system.

When we think about sex, electric signals that originate in the cerebral cortex interact with other parts of the brain and nerves, causing your heart rate to speed up and increase blood flow to our genitals.

525 billion

The number of sperm cells a male will produce over a lifetime. Roughly 68 cans of Coca-Cola worth.